TITLE: PCOS DIET COOKBOOK FOR BEGINNERS

Subtitle:A practical Guide to Managing Polycystic Ovary Syndrome through Diet and Delicious Recipes.

By

Lillian Charles

INTRODUCTION

Polycystic Ovary Syndrome (PCOS) is a common hormonal disorder that affects millions of women worldwide. It is characterized by irregular menstrual cycles, elevated levels of male hormones (androgens), and polycystic ovaries. Women with PCOS may experience a range of symptoms, including weight gain, acne, hair loss, and fertility issues. While the exact cause of PCOS is unknown, it is often linked to insulin resistance and inflammation.

Benefits of a PCOS-friendly Diet

Diet plays a crucial role in managing PCOS symptoms and improving overall health. A PCOS-friendly diet focuses on whole, nutrient-dense foods that help regulate blood sugar levels, reduce inflammation, and support hormonal balance. By making mindful food choices, you can alleviate symptoms, enhance fertility, and promote long-term wellness.

Key benefits of a PCOS-friendly diet include:

Stabilized Blood Sugar Levels: Choosing low-glycemic foods helps prevent insulin spikes and reduces the risk of developing type 2 diabetes.

Weight Management: A balanced diet rich in fiber, lean proteins, and healthy fats can support healthy weight loss and maintenance.

Reduced Inflammation: Anti-inflammatory foods can help alleviate symptoms and improve overall health.

Improved Hormonal Balance: Nutrient-dense foods provide essential vitamins and minerals that support hormonal health.

How to Use This Cookbook

This cookbook is designed to be your guide to delicious and nutritious meals that support your journey with PCOS. Whether you're new to cooking or an experienced home chef, you'll find a variety of recipes that are easy to prepare and enjoyable to eat. Each recipe includes step-by-step instructions, nutritional information, and tips for modifying dishes to suit your dietary needs.

Here's how to get the most out of this cookbook:

Start Simple: Begin with the recipes that appeal to you the most and gradually explore new dishes.

Plan Ahead: Use the meal planning tips and pantry stocking guide to make grocery shopping and meal prep more efficient.

Customize: Feel free to adapt recipes based on your preferences and dietary restrictions. Many recipes include suggestions for gluten-free, dairy-free, and vegetarian options.

Stay Informed: Refer to the sections on essential nutrients, foods to eat and avoid, and special diets for additional guidance on managing PCOS through diet.

By incorporating these recipes into your daily routine, you can take control of your health and well-being. Let's embark on this journey together and discover the transformative power of a PCOS-friendly diet!

CHAPTER ONE

Understanding PCOS and Its Impact on Diet

What is PCOS?

Polycystic Ovary Syndrome (PCOS) is a complex hormonal disorder affecting women of reproductive age. It is characterized by the presence of multiple small cysts on the ovaries, elevated levels of androgens (male hormones), and irregular menstrual cycles. PCOS can also lead to a range of symptoms and health complications, including:

Irregular periods or no periods at all

Excess hair growth (hirsutism), particularly on the face, chest, and back

Acne and oily skin

Scalp hair thinning or hair loss

Weight gain or difficulty losing weight

Insulin resistance and elevated blood sugar levels

Difficulty conceiving or infertility

Mood swings and depression

The Role of insulin resistance

A significant number of women with PCOS experience insulin resistance, a condition where the body's cells become less responsive to insulin, leading to higher levels of insulin in the blood. Insulin is a hormone that helps regulate blood sugar levels. When insulin resistance occurs, the body compensates by producing more insulin, which can exacerbate symptoms of PCOS and contribute to weight gain and increased androgen production.

The Impact of Diet on PCOS

Diet plays a crucial role in managing PCOS and its symptoms. The right diet can help regulate blood sugar levels, reduce inflammation, and support hormonal balance. Here's how diet impacts PCOS:

1.Blood Sugar Regulation:
   Consuming low-glycemic index (GI) foods helps stabilize blood sugar levels and prevents insulin spikes. Low-GI foods include whole grains, legumes, non-starchy vegetables, and certain fruits.

2.Weight Management:

A balanced diet rich in fiber, lean proteins, and healthy fats can support weight loss and maintenance. Losing even a small amount of weight can significantly improve PCOS symptoms.

3.Inflammation Reduction:

Anti-inflammatory foods, such as fatty fish, nuts, seeds, olive oil, and leafy greens, can help reduce systemic inflammation, which is often elevated in women with PCOS.

4. Hormonal Balance:

Certain nutrients, including vitamin D, B vitamins, magnesium, and omega-3 fatty acids, are essential for hormonal health. A diet rich in these nutrients can help balance hormones and improve symptoms.

Foods to Focus On

High-Fiber Foods: Whole grains, vegetables, fruits, legumes, and nuts.
Lean Proteins: Chicken, turkey, fish, tofu, legumes, and low-fat dairy.
Healthy Fats: Avocado, olive oil, nuts, seeds, and fatty fish.
Low-GI Carbohydrates: Whole grains, legumes, non-starchy vegetables, and certain fruits.

Foods to Limit or Avoid

Refined Carbohydrates: White bread, pastries, sugary snacks, and sugary beverages.

Processed Foods: Foods high in trans fats, preservatives, and artificial additives.

Sugary Foods: Sweets, candies, and desserts high in added sugars.

Dairy and Gluten: Some women with PCOS find that reducing dairy and gluten helps alleviate symptoms, though this varies from person to person.

By understanding the relationship between PCOS and diet, you can make informed choices that support your health and well-being. The following sections of this cookbook will provide you with a variety of delicious, nutrient-dense recipes designed to help you manage PCOS and enjoy a healthier lifestyle.

How Diet Affects PCOS Symptoms

Diet is a powerful tool in managing Polycystic Ovary Syndrome (PCOS) symptoms. By understanding how certain foods and nutrients impact your body, you can make dietary choices that help alleviate symptoms and improve overall health. Here are the key ways diet affects PCOS symptoms:

1. Blood Sugar Regulation

Impact on Symptoms:
Stable Blood Sugar Levels: Keeping blood sugar levels stable is crucial for managing PCOS. Sudden spikes and drops in blood sugar can worsen insulin resistance, leading to increased androgen levels and exacerbating symptoms like weight gain and hirsutism.

Reduced Insulin Resistance:A diet that emphasizes low-glycemic index (GI) foods helps prevent insulin spikes and reduces insulin resistance, a common issue in women with PCOS.

Dietary Tips:

Choose Low-GI Foods: Opt for whole grains, legumes, non-starchy vegetables, and certain fruits that digest slowly and help maintain steady blood sugar levels.

Avoid Refined Carbs and Sugars: Limit consumption of white bread, pastries, sugary snacks, and sugary beverages that cause rapid blood sugar spikes.

2. Weight Management

Impact on Symptoms:

Improved Hormonal Balance: Excess weight, particularly around the abdomen, can worsen insulin resistance and increase androgen levels. Losing even a small amount of weight can significantly improve PCOS symptoms, including menstrual regularity and fertility.

Reduced Inflammation: Weight loss can also decrease inflammation in the body, which is often elevated in women with PCOS.

Dietary Tips:

Focus on Whole Foods: Prioritize a diet rich in vegetables, fruits, lean proteins, and healthy fats.

Portion Control: Be mindful of portion sizes and avoid overeating.

3. Inflammation Reduction

Impact on Symptoms:

Lower Inflammatory Markers: Chronic inflammation is associated with many PCOS symptoms, including insulin resistance and cardiovascular issues. Anti-inflammatory foods can help lower inflammation and improve overall health.

Improved Symptom Management: Reducing inflammation can lead to better management of symptoms such as acne, fatigue, and joint pain.

Dietary Tips:

Incorporate Anti-Inflammatory Foods: Include foods like fatty fish (rich in omega-3 fatty acids), nuts, seeds, olive oil, leafy greens, and berries.

Avoid Pro-Inflammatory Foods: Limit processed foods, trans fats, and foods high in sugar and refined carbohydrates.

4. Hormonal Balance

Impact on Symptoms:
Balanced Androgen Levels: Certain nutrients play a crucial role in hormone production and regulation. Ensuring an adequate intake of these nutrients can help balance androgen levels and reduce symptoms such as acne and hirsutism.

Regular Menstrual Cycles:A balanced diet can support regular menstrual cycles and improve fertility.

Dietary Tips:

Nutrient-Rich Foods: Focus on foods high in essential nutrients such as vitamin D, B vitamins, magnesium, and omega-3 fatty acids. These include fatty fish, eggs, leafy greens, nuts, seeds, and fortified foods.

Consider Supplements: In some cases, supplements may be necessary to meet your nutritional needs, especially if you have specific deficiencies. Consult with a healthcare provider before starting any new supplements.

5. Gut Health

Impact on Symptoms:

Improved Digestion and Metabolism: A healthy gut microbiome is linked to better digestion, nutrient absorption, and metabolism. Gut health is also connected to inflammation and insulin sensitivity, both critical in managing PCOS.

Enhanced Mood and Energy Levels: A balanced gut can positively affect mood and energy levels, which are often impacted in women with PCOS.

Dietary Tips:

Probiotic and Prebiotic Foods: Include probiotic-rich foods like yogurt, kefir, and fermented vegetables, as well as prebiotic foods such as garlic, onions, bananas, and asparagus.

High-Fiber Foods: Fiber supports a healthy gut by promoting regular bowel movements and feeding beneficial gut bacteria. Incorporate a variety of vegetables, fruits, legumes, and whole grains into your diet.

By making informed dietary choices, you can manage PCOS symptoms more effectively and improve your overall quality of life. The recipes and meal plans in this cookbook are designed to support you on this journey, providing delicious and nutritious options that cater to your needs.

The Importance of a Balanced Diet for PCOS

A balanced diet is crucial for managing Polycystic Ovary Syndrome (PCOS) and improving overall health. A diet that includes a variety of nutrient-dense foods can help regulate hormones, manage weight, reduce inflammation, and stabilize blood sugar levels. Here's why a balanced diet is important and how it can benefit those with PCOS:

1. Hormonal Regulation

Why It Matters:
PCOS is characterized by hormonal imbalances, including elevated androgens (male hormones) and insulin resistance. A balanced diet can help regulate these hormones.

How It Helps:

Essential Nutrients: Vitamins and minerals such as vitamin D, B vitamins, magnesium, and omega-3 fatty acids are vital for hormone production and balance. A varied diet ensures you get these nutrients.

Healthy Fats: Incorporating healthy fats from sources like avocados, nuts, seeds, and fatty fish supports hormone production and reduces inflammation.

2. Weight Management

Why It Matters:
Many women with PCOS struggle with weight gain and find it challenging to lose weight due to insulin resistance and hormonal imbalances. Maintaining a healthy weight can alleviate many PCOS symptoms.

How It Helps:
Calorie Control:A balanced diet helps manage calorie intake, promoting weight loss or maintenance without feeling deprived.
Metabolism Boost: Eating a variety of foods ensures your body gets the nutrients it needs to function optimally, which can help improve metabolism and energy levels.

3. Blood Sugar Stability

Why It Matters:
Insulin resistance is common in women with PCOS, leading to high blood sugar levels and an increased risk of type 2 diabetes.

How It Helps:

Low-Glycemic Foods: Consuming low-glycemic index (GI) foods helps maintain steady blood sugar levels and prevents insulin spikes.

Fiber-Rich Foods: High-fiber foods, such as vegetables, fruits, legumes, and whole grains, slow the absorption of sugar into the bloodstream, aiding in blood sugar control.

4. Inflammation Reduction

Why It Matters:
Chronic inflammation is linked to many PCOS symptoms, including insulin resistance and cardiovascular issues.

How It Helps:

Anti-Inflammatory Foods: Foods like fatty fish, nuts, seeds, olive oil, leafy greens, and berries have anti-inflammatory properties that can help reduce inflammation in the body.

Avoiding Processed Foods: Limiting processed foods, trans fats, and foods high in sugar and refined carbohydrates can help decrease inflammation.

5. Improved Gut Health

Why It Matters:
A healthy gut microbiome is essential for digestion, nutrient absorption, and overall health. Gut health is also connected to inflammation and insulin sensitivity, both critical in managing PCOS.

How It Helps:

Probiotic Foods: Including probiotic-rich foods such as yogurt, kefir, and fermented vegetables supports a healthy gut microbiome.

Prebiotic Foods: Foods like garlic, onions, bananas, and asparagus feed beneficial gut bacteria, promoting gut health and function.

6. Enhanced Energy and Mood

Why It Matters:
PCOS can affect energy levels and mood, leading to fatigue and mood swings. A balanced diet provides the necessary nutrients to support mental and physical well-being.

How It Helps:

Nutrient-Dense Foods: Consuming a variety of nutrient-rich foods ensures your body gets the vitamins and minerals it needs for optimal energy production and brain function.

Regular Meals: Eating regular, balanced meals helps maintain stable blood sugar levels, preventing energy crashes and mood swings.

7. Long-Term Health

Why It Matters:
PCOS increases the risk of several long-term health conditions, including type 2 diabetes, cardiovascular disease, and metabolic syndrome.

How It Helps:

Preventative Nutrition: A balanced diet helps mitigate these risks by promoting healthy weight, stable blood sugar levels, and reduced inflammation.

Lifelong Habits: Establishing healthy eating habits early on can lead to sustained health benefits and improved quality of life.

By focusing on a balanced diet that includes a variety of whole, nutrient-dense foods, you can effectively manage PCOS symptoms and support your overall health. The recipes and meal plans in this cookbook are designed to help you achieve a balanced diet that caters to your needs and preferences.

CHAPTER TWO

Getting Started With The PCOS Diet

Key Principles of the PCOS Diet

The PCOS diet is designed to help manage the symptoms of Polycystic Ovary Syndrome (PCOS) by focusing on nutrient-dense foods that support hormonal balance, insulin regulation, and overall health. Here are the key principles to follow:

1.Low-Glycemic Index (GI) Foods

Why It Matters:
Low-GI foods help stabilize blood sugar levels and reduce insulin spikes, which is crucial for managing insulin resistance, a common issue in PCOS.

How to Implement:
Choose whole grains like quinoa, brown rice, and oats over refined grains.

Include plenty of non-starchy vegetables such as leafy greens, broccoli, and peppers.

Opt for fruits that are lower in sugar, such as berries, apples, and pears.

2.High-Fiber Foods

Why It Matters:
 High-fiber foods aid in digestion, promote a feeling of fullness, and help regulate blood sugar levels.

How to Implement:
 Incorporate plenty of vegetables, fruits, legumes, and whole grains into your diet.

 Aim for at least 25-30 grams of fiber per day.

3.Lean Proteins

Why It Matters:
 Protein helps maintain muscle mass, supports metabolic health, and can help manage weight by promoting satiety.

How to Implement:
 Include sources of lean protein such as chicken, turkey, fish, eggs, tofu, and legumes.

 Incorporate plant-based proteins like beans, lentils, and quinoa.

4.Healthy Fats

Why It Matters:
 Healthy fats are essential for hormone production and can help reduce inflammation.

How to Implement:
 Choose sources of healthy fats such as avocados, nuts, seeds, and olive oil.

 Include fatty fish like salmon, mackerel, and sardines, which are rich in omega-3 fatty acids.

5.Anti-Inflammatory Foods

Why It Matters:
 Reducing inflammation is key to managing many PCOS symptoms and improving overall health.

How to Implement:
 Focus on foods with anti-inflammatory properties such as berries, leafy greens, fatty fish, nuts, seeds, and olive oil.

 Avoid processed foods, trans fats, and foods high in sugar and refined carbohydrates.

6.Adequate Hydration

Why It Matters:
 Staying hydrated is essential for overall health, aiding in digestion, nutrient absorption, and maintaining energy levels.

How to Implement:
 Drink plenty of water throughout the day, aiming for at least 8 glasses.

Limit sugary drinks and opt for herbal teas or infused water for variety.

7. Balanced Meals

Why It Matters:
Balanced meals that include a mix of protein, healthy fats, and complex carbohydrates help maintain stable blood sugar levels and provide sustained energy.

How to Implement:
Ensure each meal contains a balance of macronutrients: protein, fat, and carbohydrates.

Include a variety of foods to ensure you're getting a wide range of nutrients.

8.Portion Control

Why It Matters:
Controlling portion sizes helps manage calorie intake, which is important for weight management and overall health.

How to Implement:
Be mindful of portion sizes and listen to your body's hunger and fullness cues.

Use smaller plates and bowls to help control portions.

9.Regular Meal Timing

Why It Matters:
 Eating regular meals helps maintain stable blood sugar levels and prevents overeating.

How to Implement:
 Aim to eat every 3-4 hours to keep your blood sugar stable.

 Plan your meals and snacks ahead of time to avoid skipping meals.

10.Mindful Eating

Why It Matters:
 Being mindful about what and how you eat can help you make healthier choices and enjoy your food more.

How to Implement:
 Eat slowly and without distractions to fully enjoy your meals and recognize when you're full.

 Pay attention to the quality of your food, choosing whole, minimally processed options whenever possible.

By adhering to these key principles, you can effectively manage PCOS symptoms and support your overall health. The recipes and meal plans provided in this cookbook are designed to help you implement these principles easily and deliciously.

Foods to Include and Avoid in a PCOS Diet

A well-planned diet is crucial for managing PCOS symptoms and improving overall health. Here's a guide on foods to include and avoid:

Foods to Include

1. Low-Glycemic Index (GI) Foods

Whole Grains: Quinoa, brown rice, oats, barley, whole wheat, bulgur

Legumes: Lentils, chickpeas, black beans, kidney beans

Non-Starchy Vegetables: Broccoli, spinach, kale, peppers, zucchini, cucumbers
Fruits: Berries, apples, pears, oranges, peaches

2. High-Fiber Foods

Vegetables: Brussels sprouts, carrots, green beans, artichokes

Fruits: Avocados, raspberries, pears, apples

Whole Grains: Oats, quinoa, barley, whole wheat

Legumes: Lentils, black beans, chickpeas

3. Lean Proteins

Poultry: Chicken, turkey

Fish: Salmon, mackerel, sardines, cod

Eggs: Whole eggs and egg whites
Plant-Based Proteins:Tofu, tempeh, edamame,
lentils

4. Healthy Fats

Avocados: Fresh avocado, avocado oil
Nuts and Seeds:Almonds, walnuts, chia seeds,
flaxseeds, pumpkin seeds

Olive Oil: Extra virgin olive oil for cooking and
dressings

Fatty Fish: Salmon, mackerel, sardines

5. Anti-Inflammatory Foods

Berries: Blueberries, strawberries, raspberries,
blackberries

Leafy Greens: Spinach, kale, Swiss chard

Nuts and Seeds: Almonds, walnuts, chia seeds, flaxseeds

Spices: Turmeric, ginger, cinnamon, garlic

6. Probiotic and Prebiotic Foods

Probiotics: Yogurt, kefir, sauerkraut, kimchi, miso, kombucha

Prebiotics: Garlic, onions, leeks, asparagus, bananas, oats

7. Hydrating Foods and Beverages

Water: Aim for at least 8 glasses a day

Herbal Teas: Green tea, chamomile tea, peppermint tea

Infused Water: Add slices of lemon, cucumber, or berries for flavor

Foods to Avoid

1. Refined Carbohydrates

White Bread and Pasta: Opt for whole grain versions instead

Pastries and Cakes: Choose homemade or healthier options with whole grains

Sugary Cereals: Select cereals high in fiber and low in added sugars

2. Sugary Foods and Beverages

Sodas and Sweetened Drinks: Drink water, herbal teas, or unsweetened beverages

Candy and Sweets: Limit intake and opt for dark chocolate or fruit for treats

Desserts: Choose healthier dessert recipes with natural sweeteners

3. Processed and Junk Foods

Fast Food: Avoid high-calorie, low-nutrient fast food options

Processed Snacks: Limit chips, crackers, and other processed snacks

Frozen Meals: Choose fresh or homemade meals over processed frozen options

4. Trans Fats and Unhealthy Fats

Fried Foods: Opt for baked or grilled versions instead

Margarine and Shortening: Use olive oil, avocado oil, or coconut oil instead

Processed Meats: Limit intake of sausages, hot dogs, and deli meats

5. Dairy and Gluten (for Some Women)

Dairy Products: Some women with PCOS find that reducing dairy helps alleviate symptoms; choose plant-based alternatives if needed

Gluten: Some women find benefit in reducing or eliminating gluten; choose gluten-free grains like quinoa, rice, and buckwheat

6. High-Sodium Foods

Processed Foods: Read labels and choose low-sodium options

Canned Soups and Vegetables: Opt for fresh or low-sodium versions

Salty Snacks: Limit intake of chips, pretzels, and salted nuts

By focusing on these foods to include and avoid, you can better manage PCOS symptoms and improve your overall health. The recipes in this cookbook will help you incorporate these principles into your daily meals.

CHAPTER THREE

Breakfast Recipes

Quick and Nutritious Breakfast Options for PCOS

Starting your day with a nutritious breakfast can help manage PCOS symptoms and provide lasting energy. Here are some quick and healthy breakfast ideas:

1.Smoothie Bowls

Ingredients:
1 cup spinach or kale
1 cup unsweetened almond milk
1 banana
1/2 cup frozen berries (blueberries, strawberries, or raspberries)
1 tablespoon chia seeds
1 tablespoon almond butter

Instructions:
Blend all ingredients until smooth.

Pour into a bowl and top with sliced fruits, nuts, and seeds.

2.Overnight Oats

Ingredients:
1/2 cup rolled oats
1/2 cup unsweetened almond milk or Greek yogurt
1 tablespoon chia seeds
1/2 teaspoon cinnamon
1/2 cup fresh or frozen berries
1 teaspoon honey or maple syrup (optional)

Instructions:
Combine oats, almond milk (or yogurt), chia seeds, and cinnamon in a jar.

Stir in berries and sweetener if using.

Cover and refrigerate overnight.

Enjoy cold or warmed up in the morning.

3.Veggie Omelet

Ingredients:
2 large eggs or egg whites
1/4 cup diced bell peppers
1/4 cup chopped spinach
1/4 cup diced tomatoes
1/4 cup diced onions
1 tablespoon olive oil or avocado oil
Salt and pepper to taste

Instructions:

Heat oil in a non-stick pan over medium heat.

Sauté vegetables until soft.

Beat eggs and pour over vegetables in the pan.

Cook until eggs are set, folding omelet in half.

Serve with a side of avocado slices.

4.Chia Seed Pudding

Ingredients:
3 tablespoons chia seeds
1 cup unsweetened almond milk
1 teaspoon vanilla extract
1 teaspoon honey or maple syrup (optional)
Fresh fruit for topping (berries, mango, or banana)

Instructions:
Mix chia seeds, almond milk, vanilla extract, and
sweetener in a bowl.

Stir well to avoid clumping.

Cover and refrigerate for at least 4 hours or
overnight.

Stir again before serving and top with fresh fruit.

5.Greek Yogurt Parfait

Ingredients:
1 cup plain Greek yogurt
1/2 cup fresh or frozen berries
1/4 cup granola (preferably low-sugar)
1 tablespoon flaxseeds or chia seeds
1 teaspoon honey (optional)

Instructions:
Layer Greek yogurt, berries, and granola in a bowl or jar.

Sprinkle with seeds and drizzle with honey if desired.

Enjoy immediately.

6.Avocado Toast

Ingredients:
1 slice whole grain or gluten-free bread
1/2 ripe avocado
1 teaspoon lemon juice
Salt and pepper to taste
Optional toppings: cherry tomatoes, radishes, sprouts, poached egg

Instructions:
Toast the bread.
Mash avocado with lemon juice, salt, and pepper.

Spread mashed avocado on toast and add optional toppings.

7.Quinoa Breakfast Bowl

Ingredients:
1/2 cup cooked quinoa
1/2 cup almond milk or other plant-based milk
1/2 banana, sliced
1 tablespoon almond butter
1 tablespoon chia seeds or flaxseeds
1/4 teaspoon cinnamon

Instructions:
Combine cooked quinoa and almond milk in a bowl.

Top with banana slices, almond butter, chia seeds, and cinnamon.

Serve warm or cold.

These breakfast options are quick to prepare, packed with nutrients, and help stabilize blood sugar levels, making them ideal for managing PCOS symptoms.

Smoothies and Shakes for Energy

Smoothies and shakes can be a quick, nutritious way to boost your energy levels, especially when dealing with PCOS. Here are some recipes designed to provide sustained energy, stabilize blood sugar levels, and support overall health.

1.Berry Blast Smoothie

Ingredients:
1 cup unsweetened almond milk
1/2 cup Greek yogurt
1 cup mixed berries (strawberries, blueberries, raspberries)
1 tablespoon chia seeds
1 tablespoon almond butter
1/2 banana

Instructions:
Combine all ingredients in a blender.

Blend until smooth.

Pour into a glass and enjoy.

2.Green Power Smoothie

Ingredients:
1 cup spinach or kale
1/2 avocado
1 cup coconut water
1/2 apple, cored and chopped
1/2 cucumber, chopped
Juice of 1/2 lemon
1 tablespoon flaxseeds

Instructions:
Place all ingredients in a blender.

Blend until smooth and creamy.

Serve immediately.

3.Protein-Packed Peanut Butter Shake

Ingredients:
1 cup unsweetened almond milk
1 scoop protein powder (preferably plant-based)
1 tablespoon natural peanut butter
1/2 banana
1 tablespoon chia seeds
1/2 teaspoon vanilla extract

Instructions:
Add all ingredients to a blender.

Blend until fully combined and smooth.

Drink up for a protein boost.

4: Tropical Mango Smoothie

Ingredients
1 cup unsweetened coconut milk
1/2 cup Greek yogurt
1 cup frozen mango chunks
1/2 banana
1 tablespoon hemp seeds

1/2 teaspoon turmeric powder

Instructions:
Combine all ingredients in a blender.

Blend until smooth.

Pour into a glass and enjoy a taste of the tropics.

5.Chocolate Banana Energy Shake

Ingredients:
1 cup unsweetened almond milk
1 scoop chocolate protein powder (preferably plant-based)
1 tablespoon cocoa powder
1 banana
1 tablespoon almond butter
1 tablespoon chia seeds

Instructions:
Place all ingredients in a blender.

Blend until smooth and creamy.

Enjoy a chocolatey treat.

6.Matcha Green Tea Smoothie

Ingredients:
1 cup unsweetened almond milk
1/2 cup Greek yogurt

1 teaspoon matcha green tea powder
1/2 banana
1/2 avocado
1 tablespoon chia seeds
1 teaspoon honey (optional)

Instructions:
Add all ingredients to a blender.

Blend until well mixed and smooth.

Drink up for an energy and antioxidant boost.

7. Berry Beet Smoothie

Ingredients:
1 cup unsweetened almond milk
1/2 cup cooked beets, chopped
1/2 cup frozen mixed berries
1/2 banana
1 tablespoon flaxseeds
1/2 teaspoon ginger powder

Instructions:
Combine all ingredients in a blender.

Blend until smooth and vibrant.

Serve immediately.

8.Oatmeal Breakfast Smoothie

Ingredients:
1 cup unsweetened almond milk
1/2 cup cooked oats
1/2 banana
1 tablespoon almond butter
1 tablespoon chia seeds
1/2 teaspoon cinnamon

Instructions:
Place all ingredients in a blender.

Blend until smooth and creamy.

Enjoy a filling and nutritious breakfast.

These smoothies and shakes are packed with essential nutrients, fiber, and healthy fats, providing a steady energy supply to help manage PCOS symptoms effectively.

CHAPTER FOUR

Lunch Recipes

Healthy and Satisfying Lunch Ideas for PCOS

A balanced and nutritious lunch can help manage PCOS symptoms and keep you energized throughout the day. Here are some healthy lunch ideas that are quick, easy, and satisfying:

1.Quinoa and Chickpea Salad

Ingredients:
1 cup cooked quinoa
1 cup canned chickpeas, drained and rinsed
1/2 cup cherry tomatoes, halved
1/2 cucumber, diced
1/4 red onion, thinly sliced
1/4 cup feta cheese, crumbled
2 tablespoons olive oil
1 tablespoon lemon juice
Salt and pepper to taste
Fresh parsley, chopped

Instructions:

In a large bowl, combine quinoa, chickpeas, cherry tomatoes, cucumber, red onion, and feta cheese.

Drizzle with olive oil and lemon juice.

Season with salt and pepper.

Toss to combine and garnish with fresh parsley.

2.Turkey and Avocado Wrap

Ingredients:
1 whole grain or gluten-free wrap
3-4 slices of roasted turkey breast
1/2 avocado, sliced
1/2 cup mixed greens
1/4 cup shredded carrots
1 tablespoon hummus

Instructions:
Spread hummus evenly over the wrap.

Layer with turkey slices, avocado, mixed greens, and shredded carrots.

Roll up the wrap tightly and cut in half.

3.Lentil and Vegetable Soup

Ingredients:
1 cup dried lentils, rinsed
1 onion, diced

2 carrots, diced
2 celery stalks, diced
3 cloves garlic, minced
1 can diced tomatoes
4 cups vegetable broth
1 teaspoon cumin
1 teaspoon paprika
Salt and pepper to taste
Fresh spinach or kale

Instructions:
In a large pot, sauté onion, carrots, celery, and garlic until softened.

Add lentils, diced tomatoes, and vegetable broth.

Stir in cumin and paprika, and season with salt and pepper.

Bring to a boil, then reduce heat and simmer for about 30 minutes, until lentils are tender.

Stir in fresh spinach or kale before serving.

4.Grilled Chicken and Veggie Bowl

Ingredients:
1 grilled chicken breast, sliced
1/2 cup cooked brown rice or quinoa
1/2 cup steamed broccoli
1/2 cup roasted sweet potatoes
1/4 cup sliced bell peppers

1 tablespoon olive oil
1 tablespoon balsamic vinegar
Salt and pepper to taste

Instructions:

Arrange brown rice or quinoa in a bowl.

Top with sliced grilled chicken, steamed broccoli, roasted sweet potatoes, and bell peppers.

Drizzle with olive oil and balsamic vinegar.

Season with salt and pepper to taste.

5.Greek Salad with Grilled Salmon

Ingredients:
1 salmon fillet
2 cups mixed greens
1/2 cup cherry tomatoes, halved
1/2 cucumber, sliced
1/4 red onion, thinly sliced
1/4 cup Kalamata olives
1/4 cup feta cheese, crumbled
2 tablespoons olive oil
1 tablespoon red wine vinegar
Salt and pepper to taste
Fresh dill or oregano

Instructions:

Grill or pan-sear the salmon fillet until cooked through.

In a large bowl, combine mixed greens, cherry tomatoes, cucumber, red onion, Kalamata olives, and feta cheese.

In a small bowl, whisk together olive oil, red wine vinegar, salt, and pepper.

Drizzle the dressing over the salad and toss to combine.

Top the salad with the grilled salmon and garnish with fresh dill or oregano.

6.Stuffed Bell Peppers

Ingredients:
4 bell peppers, tops cut off and seeds removed
1 cup cooked quinoa
1 cup black beans, drained and rinsed
1/2 cup corn kernels
1/2 cup diced tomatoes
1/4 cup chopped cilantro
1 teaspoon cumin
1 teaspoon chili powder
Salt and pepper to taste
1/2 cup shredded cheese (optional)

Instructions:
Preheat oven to 375°F (190°C).

In a large bowl, combine quinoa, black beans, corn, diced tomatoes, cilantro, cumin, chili powder, salt, and pepper.

Stuff the bell peppers with the quinoa mixture.

Place stuffed peppers in a baking dish and top with shredded cheese if using.

Bake for 25-30 minutes, until peppers are tender and cheese is melted.

7.Avocado and Tuna Salad

Ingredients:
1 can tuna, drained
1 avocado, diced
1/4 cup red onion, diced
1/4 cup celery, diced
2 tablespoons Greek yogurt or mayonnaise
1 tablespoon lemon juice
Salt and pepper to taste

Instructions:
In a bowl, combine tuna, avocado, red onion, celery, Greek yogurt or mayonnaise, and lemon juice.

Season with salt and pepper.

Mix until well combined.

Serve on a bed of mixed greens or in a whole grain wrap.

These lunch options are designed to be balanced, nutritious, and supportive of managing PCOS symptoms. They are easy to prepare and can be customized to fit your taste and dietary preferences.

Salads, Wraps, and Light Meals for PCOS

Here are some refreshing and easy-to-make options for salads, wraps, and light meals that are both healthy and satisfying.

Salads

1. Mediterranean Quinoa Salad

Ingredients:
1 cup cooked quinoa
1/2 cup cherry tomatoes, halved
1/2 cup cucumber, diced
1/4 cup red onion, thinly sliced
1/4 cup Kalamata olives, pitted and halved
1/4 cup feta cheese, crumbled
2 tablespoons olive oil

1 tablespoon red wine vinegar
1 teaspoon dried oregano
Salt and pepper to taste

Instructions:
In a large bowl, combine quinoa, cherry tomatoes, cucumber, red onion, olives, and feta cheese.

In a small bowl, whisk together olive oil, red wine vinegar, oregano, salt, and pepper.

Pour the dressing over the salad and toss to combine.

2. Spinach and Strawberry Salad

Ingredients:
2 cups fresh spinach leaves
1 cup strawberries, sliced
1/4 cup red onion, thinly sliced
1/4 cup goat cheese, crumbled
1/4 cup walnuts, toasted
2 tablespoons balsamic vinaigrette

Instructions:
In a large bowl, combine spinach, strawberries, red onion, goat cheese, and walnuts.

Drizzle with balsamic vinaigrette and toss gently to combine.

3. Chickpea and Avocado Salad

Ingredients:
1 can chickpeas, drained and rinsed
1 avocado, diced
1/2 cup cherry tomatoes, halved
1/4 cup red onion, diced
2 tablespoons fresh parsley, chopped
1 tablespoon lemon juice
2 tablespoons olive oil
Salt and pepper to taste

Instructions:
In a large bowl, combine chickpeas, avocado, cherry tomatoes, red onion, and parsley.

Drizzle with lemon juice and olive oil.

Season with salt and pepper and toss gently to combine.

Wraps

1. Hummus and Veggie Wrap

Ingredients:
1 whole grain or gluten-free wrap
2 tablespoons hummus
1/2 cup mixed greens
1/4 cup shredded carrots
1/4 cup cucumber, sliced
1/4 cup red bell pepper, sliced
1/4 avocado, sliced

Instructions:
Spread hummus evenly over the wrap.

Layer with mixed greens, shredded carrots, cucumber, bell pepper, and avocado.

Roll up the wrap tightly and cut in half.

2. Chicken Caesar Wrap

Ingredients:
1 whole grain or gluten-free wrap
1 cooked chicken breast, sliced
2 cups romaine lettuce, chopped
2 tablespoons Caesar dressing
1 tablespoon grated Parmesan cheese
1/4 cup cherry tomatoes, halved

Instructions:
In a bowl, toss romaine lettuce with Caesar dressing.

Place the lettuce mixture on the wrap and top with chicken slices, Parmesan cheese, and cherry tomatoes.

Roll up the wrap tightly and cut in half.

3. Turkey and Avocado Wrap

Ingredients:

1 whole grain or gluten-free wrap
3-4 slices roasted turkey breast
1/2 avocado, sliced
1/4 cup shredded lettuce
1/4 cup sliced cucumber
1 tablespoon Greek yogurt or mayonnaise

Instructions:
Spread Greek yogurt or mayonnaise over the wrap.

Layer with turkey slices, avocado, lettuce, and
cucumber.

Roll up the wrap tightly and cut in half.

Light Meals

1. Zucchini Noodles with Pesto

Ingredients:
2 medium zucchinis, spiralized
1/2 cup cherry tomatoes, halved
1/4 cup fresh basil pesto
2 tablespoons pine nuts, toasted
1/4 cup grated Parmesan cheese
Salt and pepper to taste

Instructions:
In a large bowl, toss zucchini noodles with basil
pesto.

Add cherry tomatoes and toss to combine.

Top with toasted pine nuts and grated Parmesan cheese.

Season with salt and pepper to taste.

2. Stuffed Bell Peppers

Ingredients:
2 bell peppers, halved and seeded
1 cup cooked quinoa
1/2 cup black beans, drained and rinsed
1/2 cup corn kernels
1/4 cup diced tomatoes
1/4 cup shredded cheese (optional)
1 tablespoon olive oil
Salt and pepper to taste

Instructions:
Preheat oven to 375°F (190°C).

In a bowl, mix quinoa, black beans, corn, diced tomatoes, olive oil, salt, and pepper.

Stuff bell pepper halves with the quinoa mixture.

Place in a baking dish and top with shredded cheese if using.

Bake for 20-25 minutes, until peppers are tender.

3. Veggie and Hummus Plate

Ingredients:
1/2 cup hummus
1 cup baby carrots
1 cup cucumber slices
1 cup bell pepper slices
1 cup cherry tomatoes
1/4 cup olives

Instructions:
Arrange baby carrots, cucumber slices, bell pepper slices, cherry tomatoes, and olives on a plate.

Serve with hummus for dipping.

These salads, wraps, and light meals are designed to be nutrient-dense, easy to prepare, and supportive of managing PCOS symptoms. Enjoy these healthy and delicious options as part of a balanced diet.

CHAPTER FIVE

Dinner Recipes

Nourishing Dinner Choices for PCOS

A balanced and nutritious dinner is essential for managing PCOS symptoms and ensuring a good night's rest. Here are some dinner ideas that are both satisfying and healthful:

1.Baked Salmon with Asparagus and Quinoa

Ingredients:
2 salmon fillets
1 bunch asparagus, trimmed
1 cup quinoa, cooked
2 tablespoons olive oil
1 lemon, sliced
2 garlic cloves, minced
Salt and pepper to taste
Fresh dill or parsley for garnish

Instructions:
Preheat oven to 400°F (200°C).

Place salmon fillets on a baking sheet lined with parchment paper.

Arrange asparagus around the salmon.

Drizzle with olive oil and sprinkle with minced garlic, salt, and pepper.

Place lemon slices on top of the salmon.

Bake for 20-25 minutes, until salmon is cooked through and asparagus is tender.

Serve with cooked quinoa and garnish with fresh dill or parsley.

2.Chicken and Vegetable Stir-Fry

Ingredients:
2 chicken breasts, thinly sliced
2 cups mixed vegetables (broccoli, bell peppers, snap peas, carrots)
2 tablespoons soy sauce or tamari
1 tablespoon sesame oil
1 tablespoon olive oil
2 garlic cloves, minced
1 tablespoon fresh ginger, minced
2 tablespoons green onions, sliced
1 tablespoon sesame seeds
Cooked brown rice or cauliflower rice for serving

Instructions:
Heat olive oil in a large skillet or wok over medium-high heat.

Add chicken slices and cook until browned and cooked through. Remove and set aside.

In the same skillet, add sesame oil, garlic, and ginger, and sauté for 1 minute.

Add mixed vegetables and stir-fry until tender-crisp, about 5-7 minutes.

Return chicken to the skillet and add soy sauce or tamari.

Stir to combine and heat through.

Serve over brown rice or cauliflower rice, garnished with green onions and sesame seeds.

3.Stuffed Bell Peppers with Ground Turkey

Ingredients:
4 bell peppers, tops cut off and seeds removed
1 pound ground turkey
1 cup cooked brown rice
1 cup tomato sauce
1 onion, diced
2 garlic cloves, minced
1 teaspoon cumin
1 teaspoon paprika
Salt and pepper to taste
1/2 cup shredded cheese (optional)
Fresh cilantro for garnish

Instructions:
Preheat oven to 375°F (190°C).

In a large skillet, cook ground turkey over medium heat until browned. Add onion and garlic and cook until softened.

Stir in cooked brown rice, tomato sauce, cumin, paprika, salt, and pepper. Cook for 5 minutes until well combined.

Stuff bell peppers with the turkey mixture and place in a baking dish.

Top with shredded cheese if using.

Bake for 25-30 minutes, until peppers are tender.

Garnish with fresh cilantro before serving.

4.Lentil and Sweet Potato Curry

Ingredients:
1 cup dried lentils, rinsed
1 large sweet potato, peeled and diced
1 onion, diced
2 garlic cloves, minced
1 tablespoon fresh ginger, minced
1 can diced tomatoes
1 can coconut milk
2 tablespoons curry powder
1 teaspoon turmeric

1 teaspoon cumin
Salt and pepper to taste
Fresh cilantro for garnish
Cooked brown rice or quinoa for serving

Instructions:
In a large pot, sauté onion, garlic, and ginger until softened.

Add curry powder, turmeric, and cumin, and cook for 1 minute.

Stir in lentils, sweet potato, diced tomatoes, and coconut milk.

Bring to a boil, then reduce heat and simmer for 25-30 minutes, until lentils and sweet potato are tender.

Season with salt and pepper.

Serve over brown rice or quinoa, garnished with fresh cilantro.

5.Vegetable and Tofu Stir-Fry

Ingredients:
1 block firm tofu, pressed and cubed
2 cups mixed vegetables (broccoli, bell peppers, carrots, snow peas)
2 tablespoons soy sauce or tamari
1 tablespoon sesame oil

1 tablespoon olive oil
2 garlic cloves, minced
1 tablespoon fresh ginger, minced
2 tablespoons green onions, sliced
1 tablespoon sesame seeds
Cooked brown rice or cauliflower rice for serving

Instructions:
Heat olive oil in a large skillet or wok over
medium-high heat.

Add tofu cubes and cook until golden brown.
Remove and set aside.

In the same skillet, add sesame oil, garlic, and
ginger, and sauté for 1 minute.

Add mixed vegetables and stir-fry until tender-crisp,
about 5-7 minutes.

Return tofu to the skillet and add soy sauce or
tamari.

Stir to combine and heat through.

Serve over brown rice or cauliflower rice, garnished
with green onions and sesame seeds.

6.Baked Cod with Lemon and Herbs

Ingredients:
2 cod fillets

2 tablespoons olive oil
1 lemon, thinly sliced
2 garlic cloves, minced
1 tablespoon fresh dill or parsley, chopped
Salt and pepper to taste
Steamed green beans or asparagus for serving

Instructions:
Preheat oven to 400°F (200°C).

Place cod fillets on a baking sheet lined with
parchment paper.

Drizzle with olive oil and sprinkle with minced garlic,
salt, and pepper.

Arrange lemon slices on top of the cod.

Bake for 15-20 minutes, until cod is opaque and
flakes easily with a fork.

Serve with steamed green beans or asparagus and
garnish with fresh dill or parsley.

7.Eggplant Parmesan

Ingredients:
1 large eggplant, sliced into rounds
1 cup marinara sauce
1 cup shredded mozzarella cheese
1/4 cup grated Parmesan cheese
1 cup almond flour

2 eggs, beaten
2 tablespoons olive oil
Fresh basil for garnish

Instructions:
Preheat oven to 375°F (190°C).

Dip eggplant slices in beaten eggs, then coat with almond flour.

Heat olive oil in a skillet over medium heat and fry eggplant slices until golden brown on both sides.

In a baking dish, spread a thin layer of marinara sauce. Layer eggplant slices on top, followed by more marinara sauce, mozzarella cheese, and Parmesan cheese.

Repeat layers until all ingredients are used, finishing with cheese on top.

Bake for 20-25 minutes, until cheese is melted and bubbly.

Garnish with fresh basil before serving.

These nourishing dinner options are designed to be balanced and nutrient-dense, helping to manage PCOS symptoms effectively while providing delicious and satisfying meals.

One-pot meals and easy dinners can save time and simplify meal preparation while ensuring you get the nutrients you need to manage PCOS symptoms. Here are some quick and delicious options:

1.One-Pot Lemon Herb Chicken and Vegetables

Ingredients:
4 chicken thighs or breasts
2 cups baby potatoes, halved
2 cups carrots, chopped
1 cup green beans, trimmed
1 lemon, sliced
2 tablespoons olive oil
3 garlic cloves, minced
1 teaspoon dried thyme
1 teaspoon dried rosemary
Salt and pepper to taste
Fresh parsley for garnish

Instructions:
Preheat oven to 400°F (200°C)
.

In a large oven-safe pot or Dutch oven, heat olive oil over medium heat.

Add chicken and cook until browned on both sides. Remove and set aside.

Add garlic to the pot and sauté for 1 minute.

Add baby potatoes, carrots, green beans, and lemon slices. Stir to combine.

Season with thyme, rosemary, salt, and pepper.

Place the chicken on top of the vegetables.

Cover the pot and bake in the oven for 25-30 minutes, until chicken is cooked through and vegetables are tender.

Garnish with fresh parsley before serving.

2.One-Pot Quinoa and Black Bean Chili

Ingredients:
1 cup quinoa, rinsed
1 can black beans, drained and rinsed
1 can diced tomatoes
1 bell pepper, chopped
1 onion, chopped
3 garlic cloves, minced
1 cup vegetable broth
2 tablespoons chili powder
1 teaspoon cumin
1 teaspoon paprika
Salt and pepper to taste
Fresh cilantro for garnish

Instructions:
In a large pot, sauté onion, bell pepper, and garlic until softened.

Add quinoa, black beans, diced tomatoes, vegetable broth, chili powder, cumin, paprika, salt, and pepper.

Bring to a boil, then reduce heat and simmer for 20-25 minutes, until quinoa is cooked and the chili has thickened.

Garnish with fresh cilantro before serving.

3. One-Pot Pasta Primavera

Ingredients:
8 oz whole grain or gluten-free pasta
2 cups broccoli florets
1 cup cherry tomatoes, halved
1 cup bell peppers, sliced
1 zucchini, sliced
3 garlic cloves, minced
2 tablespoons olive oil
4 cups vegetable broth
1/2 cup grated Parmesan cheese
1 teaspoon dried basil
1 teaspoon dried oregano
Salt and pepper to taste
Fresh basil for garnish

Instructions:

In a large pot, heat olive oil over medium heat.

Add garlic and sauté for 1 minute.

Add pasta, broccoli, cherry tomatoes, bell peppers, zucchini, vegetable broth, basil, oregano, salt, and pepper.

Bring to a boil, then reduce heat and simmer for 10-12 minutes, until pasta is cooked and vegetables are tender.

Stir in grated Parmesan cheese.

Garnish with fresh basil before serving.

4.One-Pot Moroccan Chickpea Stew

Ingredients:
1 can chickpeas, drained and rinsed
1 sweet potato, peeled and diced
1 carrot, chopped
1 onion, chopped
3 garlic cloves, minced
1 can diced tomatoes
2 cups vegetable broth
1 teaspoon cumin
1 teaspoon coriander
1 teaspoon cinnamon
1/2 teaspoon turmeric
Salt and pepper to taste
Fresh cilantro for garnish

Cooked brown rice or quinoa for serving

Instructions:
In a large pot, sauté onion, carrot, and garlic until
softened.

Add sweet potato, chickpeas, diced tomatoes,
vegetable broth, cumin, coriander, cinnamon,
turmeric, salt, and pepper.

Bring to a boil, then reduce heat and simmer for
20-25 minutes, until vegetables are tender.

Serve over brown rice or quinoa, garnished with
fresh cilantro.

5.One-Pot Chicken and Rice

Ingredients:
4 chicken thighs or breasts
1 cup brown rice
2 cups chicken broth
1 onion, chopped
2 garlic cloves, minced
1 bell pepper, chopped
1 cup frozen peas
2 tablespoons olive oil
1 teaspoon paprika
1 teaspoon dried thyme
Salt and pepper to taste
Fresh parsley for garnish

Instructions:
In a large pot, heat olive oil over medium heat.

Add chicken and cook until browned on both sides. Remove and set aside.

Add onion, bell pepper, and garlic to the pot and sauté until softened.

Stir in brown rice, chicken broth, paprika, thyme, salt, and pepper.

Place chicken on top of the rice mixture.

Cover the pot and simmer for 25-30 minutes, until chicken is cooked through and rice is tender.

Stir in frozen peas and cook for an additional 5 minutes.

Garnish with fresh parsley before serving.

6.One-Pot Shrimp and Vegetable Paella

Ingredients:
1 pound shrimp, peeled and deveined
1 cup brown rice
2 cups vegetable or chicken broth
1 bell pepper, chopped
1 cup peas
1 tomato, chopped
1 onion, chopped

3 garlic cloves, minced
2 tablespoons olive oil
1 teaspoon smoked paprika
1/2 teaspoon turmeric
Salt and pepper to taste
Fresh parsley for garnish

Instructions:
In a large pot, heat olive oil over medium heat.

Add onion, bell pepper, and garlic and sauté until softened.

Stir in brown rice, broth, smoked paprika, turmeric, salt, and pepper.

Bring to a boil, then reduce heat and simmer for 20 minutes.

Add shrimp, peas, and tomato.

Cover and cook for an additional 5-7 minutes, until shrimp are cooked through and rice is tender.

Garnish with fresh parsley before serving.

These one-pot meals and easy dinners are designed to be quick, nutritious, and supportive of managing PCOS symptoms while minimizing cleanup and preparation time.

CHAPTER SIX

Snacks and Appetizers

Snack Ideas to Keep You Energized

Maintaining steady energy levels throughout the day is essential, especially for managing PCOS. Here are some snack ideas that are nutritious, easy to prepare, and great for keeping you energized.

1.Greek Yogurt with Berries and Nuts

Ingredients:
1 cup Greek yogurt
1/2 cup mixed berries (blueberries, strawberries, raspberries)
2 tablespoons chopped nuts (almonds, walnuts, pecans)

Instructions:
Combine Greek yogurt with mixed berries.

Sprinkle with chopped nuts for added crunch and protein.

2.Apple Slices with Almond Butter

Ingredients:
1 apple, sliced

2 tablespoons almond butter

Instructions:
Slice the apple into thin wedges.

Serve with almond butter for dipping.

3.Hummus and Veggie Sticks

Ingredients:
1/2 cup hummus
1 cup assorted veggie sticks (carrots, celery,
cucumber, bell peppers)

Instructions:
Arrange veggie sticks on a plate.

Serve with hummus for dipping.

4.Energy Balls

Ingredients:
1 cup rolled oats
1/2 cup peanut butter or almond butter
1/4 cup honey or maple syrup
1/4 cup dark chocolate chips or raisins
1/4 cup chia seeds or flax seeds

Instructions:
In a large bowl, combine all ingredients and mix
well.

Roll mixture into small balls.

Store in the refrigerator for up to a week.

5.Trail Mix

Ingredients:
1/2 cup mixed nuts (almonds, cashews, walnuts)
1/4 cup dried fruit (raisins, cranberries, apricots)
1/4 cup dark chocolate chips
2 tablespoons sunflower seeds or pumpkin seeds

Instructions:
Mix all ingredients together in a bowl.

Store in an airtight container for a quick and easy snack.

6.Avocado Toast

Ingredients:
1 slice whole grain or gluten-free bread, toasted
1/2 avocado, mashed
Salt and pepper to taste
Optional toppings: cherry tomatoes, radishes, red pepper flakes

Instructions:
Spread mashed avocado on the toast.

Season with salt and pepper.

Add optional toppings as desired.

7.Cottage Cheese with Pineapple

Ingredients:
1 cup cottage cheese
1/2 cup pineapple chunks (fresh or canned in juice)

Instructions:
Combine cottage cheese with pineapple chunks for a sweet and savory snack.

8. Edamame

Ingredients:
1 cup edamame (fresh or frozen)
Salt to taste

Instructions:
Steam or microwave edamame until tender.

Sprinkle with salt and enjoy warm or chilled.

9.Hard-Boiled Eggs

Ingredients:
2 hard-boiled eggs
Salt and pepper to taste

Instructions:
Boil eggs, peel, and season with salt and pepper for a protein-packed snack.

10.Smoothie

Ingredients:
1 cup unsweetened almond milk or other
plant-based milk
1/2 banana
1/2 cup spinach
1/2 cup frozen berries
1 tablespoon chia seeds or flax seeds

Instructions:
Blend all ingredients until smooth.

Pour into a glass and enjoy immediately.

These snacks are designed to provide a balance of
protein, healthy fats, and fiber, keeping you
energized and satisfied between meals.

Appetizers for Parties and Gatherings

Having delicious and healthy appetizers at your
parties and gatherings can impress your guests
while keeping the options nutritious. Here are some
appetizer ideas that are both tasty and suitable for
managing PCOS:

1.Stuffed Mini Bell Peppers

Ingredients:
12 mini bell peppers, halved and seeded
1 cup hummus
1/4 cup crumbled feta cheese
2 tablespoons chopped fresh parsley

Instructions:
Fill each mini bell pepper half with hummus.

Top with crumbled feta cheese and sprinkle with fresh parsley.

2.Cucumber and Smoked Salmon Bites

Ingredients:
1 cucumber, sliced into rounds
4 ounces smoked salmon, cut into small pieces
1/4 cup cream cheese or Greek yogurt
1 tablespoon fresh dill, chopped
1 tablespoon capers

Instructions:
Spread a small amount of cream cheese or Greek yogurt on each cucumber slice.

Top with a piece of smoked salmon, a sprinkle of dill, and a few capers.

3.Caprese Skewers

Ingredients:
1 cup cherry tomatoes

1 cup mozzarella balls (bocconcini)
Fresh basil leaves
Balsamic glaze

Instructions:
Thread a cherry tomato, a basil leaf, and a
mozzarella ball onto small skewers or toothpicks.

Drizzle with balsamic glaze before serving.

4.Avocado Deviled Eggs

Ingredients:
6 hard-boiled eggs, halved and yolks removed
1 avocado, mashed
1 tablespoon lime juice
1 teaspoon Dijon mustard
Salt and pepper to taste
Paprika for garnish

Instructions:
In a bowl, mash egg yolks with avocado, lime juice,
Dijon mustard, salt, and pepper until smooth.

Spoon the mixture into the egg white halves.

Sprinkle with paprika before serving.

5.Baked Zucchini Chips

Ingredients:
2 zucchinis, thinly sliced

2 tablespoons olive oil
1/2 teaspoon salt
1/2 teaspoon black pepper
1/2 teaspoon garlic powder

Instructions:
Preheat oven to 425°F (220°C).

Toss zucchini slices with olive oil, salt, pepper, and garlic powder.

Arrange in a single layer on a baking sheet lined with parchment paper.

Bake for 15-20 minutes, until crispy and golden.

6.Shrimp Cocktail

Ingredients:
1 pound cooked shrimp, peeled and deveined
1 cup cocktail sauce
1 lemon, cut into wedges

Instructions:
Arrange shrimp on a platter with a bowl of cocktail sauce in the center.

Garnish with lemon wedges and serve chilled.

7.Bruschetta

Ingredients:

1 baguette, sliced into rounds
2 cups cherry tomatoes, diced
1/4 cup fresh basil, chopped
2 garlic cloves, minced
2 tablespoons balsamic vinegar
2 tablespoons olive oil
Salt and pepper to taste

Instructions:
Preheat oven to 375°F (190°C).

Toast baguette slices in the oven until lightly golden.

In a bowl, combine cherry tomatoes, basil, garlic, balsamic vinegar, olive oil, salt, and pepper.

Spoon tomato mixture onto toasted baguette slices and serve.

8.Guacamole and Veggie Platter

Ingredients:
3 avocados, mashed
1/2 cup diced tomatoes
1/4 cup diced red onion
1 tablespoon lime juice
2 garlic cloves, minced
Salt and pepper to taste
Assorted veggie sticks (carrots, celery, bell peppers, cucumber)

Instructions:
In a bowl, combine mashed avocados, tomatoes, red onion, lime juice, garlic, salt, and pepper.

Serve guacamole with a platter of assorted veggie sticks.

9.Spinach and Artichoke Dip

Ingredients:
1 can artichoke hearts, drained and chopped
1 cup frozen spinach, thawed and drained
1/2 cup Greek yogurt
1/2 cup grated Parmesan cheese
1/2 cup shredded mozzarella cheese
2 garlic cloves, minced
Salt and pepper to taste

Instructions:
Preheat oven to 375°F (190°C).

In a bowl, mix artichoke hearts, spinach, Greek yogurt, Parmesan cheese, mozzarella cheese, garlic, salt, and pepper.

Transfer the mixture to a baking dish and bake for 20 minutes, until bubbly and golden.

Serve warm with whole grain crackers or veggie sticks.

10.Roasted Chickpeas

Ingredients:
1 can chickpeas, drained and rinsed
2 tablespoons olive oil
1 teaspoon paprika
1/2 teaspoon cumin
1/2 teaspoon garlic powder
Salt and pepper to taste

Instructions:
Preheat oven to 400°F (200°C).

Toss chickpeas with olive oil, paprika, cumin, garlic powder, salt, and pepper.

Spread chickpeas on a baking sheet and roast for 20-25 minutes, until crispy.

Let cool slightly before serving.

These appetizers are not only delicious but also packed with nutrients to keep your guests satisfied and energized throughout the event.

CHAPTER SEVEN

Dessert and Treats

Guilt-Free Desserts for PCOS

Indulging in sweet treats doesn't have to derail your efforts to manage PCOS. Here are some delicious, guilt-free dessert options that are both satisfying and supportive of your health goals.

1.Chia Seed Pudding

Ingredients:
1/4 cup chia seeds
1 cup unsweetened almond milk or coconut milk
1 tablespoon maple syrup or honey
1/2 teaspoon vanilla extract
Fresh berries or nuts for topping

Instructions:
In a bowl, mix chia seeds, almond milk, maple syrup, and vanilla extract.

Stir well and let sit for 5 minutes, then stir again to prevent clumping.

Cover and refrigerate for at least 2 hours or overnight.

Top with fresh berries or nuts before serving.

2.Baked Apples with Cinnamon

Ingredients:
4 apples, cored and sliced
1 teaspoon cinnamon
2 tablespoons chopped nuts (walnuts, almonds)
1 tablespoon coconut oil or butter, melted
1 tablespoon honey or maple syrup

Instructions:
Preheat oven to 375°F (190°C).

Place apple slices in a baking dish.

Sprinkle with cinnamon, nuts, and drizzle with melted coconut oil and honey.

Bake for 25-30 minutes, until apples are tender.

Serve warm.

3.Dark Chocolate Avocado Mousse

Ingredients:
2 ripe avocados
1/4 cup unsweetened cocoa powder
1/4 cup maple syrup or honey

1/4 cup unsweetened almond milk
1 teaspoon vanilla extract
Pinch of salt

Instructions:
In a food processor, blend avocados until smooth.

Add cocoa powder, maple syrup, almond milk,
vanilla extract, and salt.

Blend until creamy and smooth.

Chill in the refrigerator for at least 30 minutes
before serving.

4.Berry Greek Yogurt Parfait

Ingredients:
1 cup Greek yogurt
1 cup mixed berries (blueberries, strawberries,
raspberries)
1 tablespoon honey or maple syrup
1/4 cup granola (optional)

Instructions:
Layer Greek yogurt, berries, and honey in a glass
or bowl.

Top with granola if desired.

Serve immediately.

5.Coconut Macaroons

Ingredients:
2 cups unsweetened shredded coconut
1/4 cup almond flour
1/4 cup maple syrup or honey
2 egg whites
1 teaspoon vanilla extract
Pinch of salt

Instructions:
Preheat oven to 350°F (175°C).

In a bowl, mix shredded coconut, almond flour,
maple syrup, egg whites, vanilla extract, and salt
until well combined.

Scoop tablespoon-sized mounds onto a baking
sheet lined with parchment paper.

Bake for 15-20 minutes, until golden brown.

Let cool before serving.

6.Frozen Banana Bites

Ingredients:
2 bananas, sliced
1/2 cup dark chocolate chips
1 tablespoon coconut oil
1/4 cup chopped nuts (optional)

Instructions:
Line a baking sheet with parchment paper.

Place banana slices on the baking sheet and freeze
for 1 hour.

In a microwave-safe bowl, melt dark chocolate
chips and coconut oil in 30-second intervals, stirring
in between.

Dip frozen banana slices in melted chocolate and
place back on the parchment paper.

Sprinkle with chopped nuts if desired.
Freeze for another 30 minutes before serving.

7.Almond Flour Brownies

Ingredients:
1 cup almond flour
1/4 cup unsweetened cocoa powder
1/2 teaspoon baking soda
1/4 teaspoon salt
1/4 cup coconut oil, melted
1/4 cup maple syrup or honey
2 eggs
1 teaspoon vanilla extract
1/2 cup dark chocolate chips

Instructions:
Preheat oven to 350°F (175°C).

In a bowl, mix almond flour, cocoa powder, baking soda, and salt.

In another bowl, whisk together melted coconut oil, maple syrup, eggs, and vanilla extract.

Combine wet and dry ingredients until smooth.

Fold in dark chocolate chips.

Pour batter into a greased 8x8 inch baking pan.

Bake for 20-25 minutes, until a toothpick inserted into the center comes out clean.

Let cool before cutting into squares.

8.Raspberry Chia Jam Bars

Ingredients:
1 1/2 cups almond flour
1/2 cup coconut flour
1/2 cup coconut oil, melted
1/4 cup maple syrup or honey
1 teaspoon vanilla extract
1 1/2 cups fresh or frozen raspberries
2 tablespoons chia seeds

Instructions:
Preheat oven to 350°F (175°C).

In a bowl, mix almond flour, coconut flour, melted coconut oil, maple syrup, and vanilla extract until a dough forms.

Press 2/3 of the dough into a greased 8x8 inch baking pan.

In a saucepan, cook raspberries over medium heat until they break down and become saucy.

Stir in chia seeds and cook for another 2 minutes.

Spread raspberry chia jam over the dough in the baking pan.

Crumble the remaining dough over the jam layer.

Bake for 25-30 minutes, until the top is golden brown.

Let cool before cutting into bars.

These guilt-free desserts are perfect for satisfying your sweet tooth while staying mindful of your PCOS management goals.

Sweet Treats Without Compromising Health

Here are some healthy and delicious sweet treat options that cater to PCOS management, ensuring you can enjoy your desserts guilt-free:

1. Greek Yogurt with Honey and Nuts

Ingredients:
1 cup Greek yogurt
1 tablespoon honey
2 tablespoons chopped nuts (walnuts, almonds, pistachios)

Instructions:
Spoon Greek yogurt into a bowl.

Drizzle with honey and sprinkle with chopped nuts.

2. Baked Pears with Cinnamon

Ingredients:
2 pears, halved and cored
1 tablespoon honey or maple syrup
1 teaspoon cinnamon
2 tablespoons chopped walnuts

Instructions:
Preheat oven to 375°F (190°C).

Place pear halves in a baking dish.

Drizzle with honey and sprinkle with cinnamon and walnuts.

Bake for 20-25 minutes, until pears are tender.

3.Chocolate-Dipped Strawberries

Ingredients:
1 cup fresh strawberries
1/2 cup dark chocolate chips
1 tablespoon coconut oil

Instructions:
In a microwave-safe bowl, melt dark chocolate chips and coconut oil in 30-second intervals, stirring in between.

Dip each strawberry into the melted chocolate and place on a parchment-lined baking sheet.

Refrigerate until chocolate is set.

4.Oatmeal Raisin Cookies

Ingredients:
1 cup rolled oats
1/2 cup almond flour
1/4 cup coconut oil, melted
1/4 cup maple syrup or honey
1/4 cup raisins
1 teaspoon vanilla extract
1/2 teaspoon cinnamon
1/4 teaspoon baking soda
Pinch of salt

Instructions:
Preheat oven to 350°F (175°C).

In a bowl, mix all ingredients until well combined.

Scoop tablespoon-sized balls onto a baking sheet
lined with parchment paper.
Flatten slightly with a fork.

Bake for 10-12 minutes, until golden brown.

Let cool before serving.

5. Berry Chia Jam

Ingredients:
2 cups mixed berries (fresh or frozen)
2 tablespoons chia seeds
1-2 tablespoons honey or maple syrup (optional)
1 teaspoon lemon juice

Instructions:
In a saucepan, cook berries over medium heat until
they break down and become saucy.

Stir in chia seeds, honey (if using), and lemon juice.

Cook for another 5 minutes, stirring frequently.

Remove from heat and let cool.

Store in an airtight container in the refrigerator.

6.Almond Butter Banana Bites

Ingredients:
2 bananas, sliced
1/4 cup almond butter
1/4 cup dark chocolate chips
1 tablespoon coconut oil

Instructions:
Place banana slices on a parchment-lined baking sheet.

Spread a small amount of almond butter on half of the banana slices.

Top with the remaining banana slices to create sandwiches.

In a microwave-safe bowl, melt dark chocolate chips and coconut oil in 30-second intervals, stirring in between.

Dip each banana sandwich into the melted chocolate and place back on the baking sheet.

Freeze for 1 hour before serving.

7.Apple Nachos

Ingredients:

2 apples, thinly sliced
2 tablespoons almond butter or peanut butter
1 tablespoon dark chocolate chips, melted
1 tablespoon chopped nuts (optional)
1 tablespoon unsweetened coconut flakes
(optional)

Instructions:
Arrange apple slices on a plate.

Drizzle with almond butter and melted dark
chocolate.

Sprinkle with chopped nuts and coconut flakes if
desired.

8.Coconut Milk Ice Cream

Ingredients:
1 can full-fat coconut milk
1/4 cup honey or maple syrup
1 teaspoon vanilla extract
1/2 cup fresh or frozen berries (optional)

Instructions:
In a bowl, whisk together coconut milk, honey, and
vanilla extract until smooth.

Pour mixture into an ice cream maker and churn
according to the manufacturer's instructions.

If using berries, add them in the last 5 minutes of churning.

Transfer to a container and freeze until firm.

9.Pumpkin Spice Energy Balls

Ingredients:
1 cup rolled oats
1/4 cup pumpkin puree
1/4 cup almond butter
1/4 cup honey or maple syrup
1 teaspoon pumpkin pie spice
1/4 cup dark chocolate chips

Instructions:
In a bowl, mix all ingredients until well combined.

Roll mixture into small balls.

Store in the refrigerator for up to a week.

10.Frozen Yogurt Bark

Ingredients:
2 cups Greek yogurt
1-2 tablespoons honey or maple syrup
1/2 cup mixed berries
1/4 cup chopped nuts
1/4 cup unsweetened coconut flakes

Instructions:

Line a baking sheet with parchment paper.

In a bowl, mix Greek yogurt and honey.

Spread yogurt mixture evenly on the baking sheet.

Sprinkle with mixed berries, nuts, and coconut
flakes.

Freeze for 2-3 hours, until firm.

Break into pieces and store in the freezer.

These sweet treats provide a healthy balance of
nutrients and flavors, allowing you to enjoy dessert
without compromising your health or PCOS
management.

CHAPTER EIGHT

Beverages and Drinks

Refreshing Drink Options

Staying hydrated and enjoying refreshing beverages is important, especially when managing PCOS. Here are some healthy and delicious drink options:

1. Infused Water

Ingredients:
1 pitcher of water
Slices of cucumber, lemon, lime, or orange
Fresh mint leaves

Instructions:
Add fruit slices and mint leaves to the pitcher of water.

Let it sit in the refrigerator for at least 1 hour before serving.

2.Green Tea Lemonade

Ingredients:
2 cups brewed green tea, chilled
1 cup fresh lemon juice

2 tablespoons honey or maple syrup
3 cups cold water
Ice cubes

Instructions:
In a pitcher, mix chilled green tea, lemon juice,
honey, and cold water.

Stir well and serve over ice.

3. Berry Smoothie

Ingredients:
1 cup unsweetened almond milk
1/2 cup mixed berries (fresh or frozen)
1/2 banana
1 tablespoon chia seeds or flaxseeds
1 teaspoon honey or maple syrup (optional)

Instructions:
Blend all ingredients until smooth.

Pour into a glass and serve immediately.

4.Coconut Water and Pineapple Cooler

Ingredients:
1 cup coconut water
1/2 cup pineapple juice
Juice of 1 lime
Ice cubes

Instructions:
Mix coconut water, pineapple juice, and lime juice in a glass.

Serve over ice.

5. Herbal Iced Tea

Ingredients:
4 herbal tea bags (chamomile, peppermint, or hibiscus)
4 cups boiling water
2 tablespoons honey or maple syrup
4 cups cold water
Ice cubes
Lemon slices or fresh herbs for garnish

Instructions:
Steep tea bags in boiling water for 5-10 minutes.

Remove tea bags and stir in honey.

Let cool to room temperature, then add cold water.

Serve over ice with lemon slices or fresh herbs.

6.Mango Lassi

Ingredients:
1 cup plain Greek yogurt
1 cup diced fresh or frozen mango
1/2 cup unsweetened almond milk

1 tablespoon honey or maple syrup
1/4 teaspoon ground cardamom (optional)
Ice cubes

Instructions:
Blend all ingredients until smooth.

Pour into a glass and serve immediately.

7.Watermelon Mint Cooler

Ingredients:
2 cups diced watermelon
1/2 cup cold water
Juice of 1 lime
Fresh mint leaves
Ice cubes

Instructions:
Blend watermelon, cold water, and lime juice until smooth.

Serve over ice with fresh mint leaves.

8Cucumber Mint Sparkler

Ingredients:
1/2 cucumber, thinly sliced
Fresh mint leaves
Juice of 1 lemon
Sparkling water
Ice cubes

Instructions:
In a glass, add cucumber slices, mint leaves, and lemon juice.

Top with sparkling water and ice.

9.Golden Milk

Ingredients:
1 cup unsweetened almond milk
1/2 teaspoon turmeric powder
1/4 teaspoon ground cinnamon
1/4 teaspoon ground ginger
1 tablespoon honey or maple syrup
Pinch of black pepper

Instructions:
In a small saucepan, warm almond milk over medium heat.

Whisk in turmeric, cinnamon, ginger, honey, and black pepper.

Heat until just hot (do not boil).

Pour into a mug and serve.

10.Iced Matcha Latte

Ingredients:
1 teaspoon matcha powder

1/4 cup hot water
1 cup unsweetened almond milk
1 tablespoon honey or maple syrup (optional)
Ice cubes

Instructions:
In a small bowl, whisk matcha powder with hot water until smooth.

Fill a glass with ice cubes.

Pour almond milk into the glass, then stir in the matcha mixture.

Sweeten with honey if desired.

These refreshing drink options are not only hydrating but also packed with nutrients that can support your overall health and well-being.

PCOS-Friendly Beverages

Managing PCOS involves making dietary choices that support hormone balance, blood sugar control, and overall health. Here are some beverage options that can help:

1.Cinnamon Spice Tea

Cinnamon helps regulate blood sugar levels and has anti-inflammatory properties.

Ingredients:
1 cinnamon stick or 1 teaspoon ground cinnamon
2 cups boiling water
Honey or stevia (optional)

Instructions:
Steep the cinnamon stick or ground cinnamon in boiling water for 10 minutes.

Strain and sweeten if desired.

2. Apple Cider Vinegar Drink
Apple cider vinegar can help improve insulin sensitivity.

Ingredients:
1 tablespoon apple cider vinegar
1 cup water
1 teaspoon honey or stevia (optional)
Ice cubes

Instructions:
Mix apple cider vinegar with water.

Sweeten if desired and serve over ice.

3.Turmeric Latte (Golden Milk)
Turmeric has anti-inflammatory and antioxidant properties.

Ingredients:
1 cup unsweetened almond milk
1/2 teaspoon turmeric powder
1/4 teaspoon ground cinnamon
1/4 teaspoon ground ginger
1 tablespoon honey or maple syrup
Pinch of black pepper

Instructions:
Warm almond milk in a saucepan over medium heat.

Whisk in turmeric, cinnamon, ginger, honey, and black pepper.

Heat until hot but not boiling. Serve warm.

4.Green Smoothie

Leafy greens are packed with nutrients that support hormone balance.

Ingredients:
1 cup unsweetened almond milk or coconut water
1 cup spinach or kale
1/2 banana
1/2 cup pineapple chunks
1 tablespoon chia seeds or flaxseeds

Instructions:
Blend all ingredients until smooth. Serve immediately.

5.Peppermint Tea

Peppermint can help reduce androgen levels in women with PCOS.

Ingredients:

1 peppermint tea bag or 1 tablespoon fresh peppermint leaves
1 cup boiling water

Instructions:

Steep tea bag or peppermint leaves in boiling water for 5-10 minutes.

Strain and serve.

6.Berry Infused Water

Berries are rich in antioxidants and have a low glycemic index.

Ingredients:

1 cup mixed berries (strawberries, blueberries, raspberries)
1 pitcher of water

Instructions:

Add berries to the pitcher of water.

Let sit in the refrigerator for at least 1 hour before serving.

7.Lemon Ginger Water

Ginger helps with digestion and inflammation, while lemon is detoxifying.

Ingredients:
1-inch piece of fresh ginger, sliced
Juice of 1 lemon
1 pitcher of water

Instructions:
Add ginger slices and lemon juice to the pitcher of water.

Let sit in the refrigerator for at least 1 hour before serving.

8.Matcha Green Tea
Matcha is rich in antioxidants and can help boost metabolism.

Ingredients:
1 teaspoon matcha powder
1/4 cup hot water
1 cup unsweetened almond milk
1 teaspoon honey or stevia (optional)
Ice cubes

Instructions:
Whisk matcha powder with hot water until smooth.

Fill a glass with ice cubes.

Pour almond milk into the glass, then stir in the matcha mixture.

Sweeten if desired.

9.Chia Fresca

Chia seeds are high in fiber and can help with satiety and blood sugar control.

Ingredients:

1 cup water or coconut water
1 tablespoon chia seeds
Juice of 1 lemon or lime
Honey or stevia (optional)

Instructions:

Mix all ingredients in a glass.

Let sit for 10 minutes to allow chia seeds to expand, stirring occasionally. Serve chilled.

10.Herbal Infusions

Various herbal teas can support different aspects of PCOS management.

Ingredients:

Choose from spearmint, chamomile, dandelion root, or nettle tea bags or loose herbs
1 cup boiling water

Instructions:

Steep the chosen tea bag or herbs in boiling water for 5-10 minutes.

Strain and serve.

These PCOS-friendly beverages provide a variety of nutrients and benefits to support hormone balance, reduce inflammation, and help manage blood sugar levels.

CHAPTER TEN

Meals Planning and Preparation Tips

How to Plan Meals for the Week

Planning meals for the week can streamline your routine, save time, and help you stay on track with your dietary goals, especially when managing PCOS. Here's a step-by-step guide to effective meal planning:

1.Set Your Goals

Identify Your Needs: Consider your nutritional needs, dietary preferences, and any specific goals related to PCOS management (e.g., low glycemic index, anti-inflammatory foods).

Decide on Meals: Determine how many breakfasts, lunches, dinners, and snacks you need to plan for.

2.Create a Weekly Menu

Choose Your Recipes: Select recipes that align with your goals and preferences. Include a variety of proteins, vegetables, and healthy fats.

Plan Balanced Meals: Ensure each meal includes a good balance of protein, healthy fats, and complex carbohydrates.

3.Make a Shopping List

List Ingredients: Write down all the ingredients you need for your weekly recipes.

Check Your Pantry: Before shopping, check what you already have to avoid buying duplicates.

4.Prepare a Cooking Schedule

Designate Cooking Days: Choose specific days for meal prep and cooking. This might be a few hours on the weekend or a couple of evenings during the week.

Batch Cooking: Prepare larger quantities of meals that can be stored and reheated throughout the week (e.g., soups, stews, grains).

5.Portion and Store

Portion Meals: Divide cooked meals into individual portions for easy access. Use airtight containers to keep food fresh.

Label and Date: Label containers with the date and meal name to keep track of freshness.

6.Incorporate Flexibility

Allow for Changes: Be flexible with your plan in case you need to adjust due to changes in schedule or availability of ingredients.

Include Quick Options: Have a few quick and easy meal options for busy days (e.g., salads, wraps).

7. Track and Evaluate

Review Your Plan: At the end of the week, review what worked well and what didn't.

Adjust as Needed: Make adjustments based on your experience and any changes in your needs or preferences.

Sample Weekly Meal Plan

Monday:

Breakfast: Greek yogurt with berries and nuts
Lunch: Quinoa salad with chickpeas, cucumber, and feta
Dinner: Baked salmon with roasted sweet potatoes and broccoli
Snack: Apple slices with almond butter

Tuesday:

Breakfast: Chia seed pudding with almond milk and strawberries
Lunch: Turkey and avocado wrap with a side of carrot sticks

Dinner: Stir-fried tofu with mixed vegetables and brown rice
Snack: Handful of mixed nuts

Wednesday:

Breakfast: Smoothie with spinach, banana, and almond milk
Lunch: Lentil soup with a side of mixed greens
Dinner: Stuffed bell peppers with quinoa and black beans
Snack: Greek yogurt with a drizzle of honey

Thursday:

Breakfast: Oatmeal with walnuts and blueberries
Lunch: Grilled chicken salad with avocado and olive oil dressing
Dinner: Spaghetti squash with marinara sauce and a side salad
Snack: Celery sticks with hummus

Friday:

Breakfast: Avocado toast on whole-grain bread
Lunch: Chickpea and vegetable curry with a side of brown rice
Dinner: Baked chicken breast with steamed green beans and sweet potato
Snack: Cottage cheese with sliced peaches

Saturday:

Breakfast: Scrambled eggs with spinach and tomatoes
Lunch: Tuna salad with mixed greens and a side of quinoa
Dinner: Turkey meatballs with roasted vegetables
Snack: Smoothie with kale, pineapple, and coconut water

Sunday:

Breakfast: Overnight oats with chia seeds and raspberries
Lunch: Mediterranean chickpea salad with a side of whole-grain pita
Dinner: Grilled shrimp with cauliflower rice and sautéed zucchini
Snack: Sliced bell peppers with guacamole

This plan helps you stay organized and ensures you're consistently eating meals that support your health goals.

Tips for Efficient Meal Preparation

1.Plan Ahead

Create a Weekly Menu: Plan your meals and snacks for the week, including recipes and portion sizes.

Make a Shopping List: List all ingredients needed for your meals to streamline grocery shopping.

2.Batch Cooking

Cook in Bulk: Prepare large quantities of staples like grains (quinoa, rice), proteins (chicken, tofu), and vegetables.

Use Freezer-Friendly Recipes: Make and freeze meals like soups, stews, and casseroles for easy access.

3.Prep Ingredients in Advance

Chop Vegetables: Wash, peel, and chop vegetables for easy access during the week.

Pre-cook Proteins: Grill, bake, or sauté proteins in advance and store in the refrigerator or freezer.

4.Utilize Kitchen Gadgets

Slow Cooker or Instant Pot: Use these appliances for easy, hands-off meal preparation.

Food Processor: Speed up chopping and blending tasks.

5.Organize Your Kitchen

Use Clear Containers: Store prepped ingredients and meals in clear, labeled containers for easy identification.

Keep a Clean Workspace: Maintain an organized kitchen to streamline cooking and clean-up.

6.Follow a Routine

Set a Prep Day: Designate a specific day and time each week for meal prep (e.g., Sunday afternoons).

Stick to a Schedule: Prepare ingredients or meals according to your weekly plan to stay on track.

7.Portion Control

Use Containers with Dividers: Portion out meals into containers with compartments to control serving sizes.

Measure Ingredients: Use measuring cups and spoons to ensure accurate portion sizes.

8. Quick Cooking Techniques

Stir-fry: Cook vegetables and proteins quickly in a hot pan for a fast, nutritious meal.

Sheet Pan Meals: Roast multiple ingredients on a single sheet pan for easy prep and clean-up.

9.Stay Flexible

Prepare Versatile Ingredients: Cook ingredients that can be used in multiple dishes (e.g., grilled chicken for salads and wraps).

Use Leftovers Creatively: Repurpose leftovers into new meals, such as turning roasted vegetables into soups or stews.

10.Clean as You Go

Minimize Clean-Up: Wash dishes, utensils, and surfaces while you cook to avoid a pile-up of dishes later.

By incorporating these tips, you can make meal preparation more efficient and enjoyable, ensuring you stick to your dietary goals and save time throughout the week.

CHAPTER TEN

Lifestyle Tips for Managing PCOS

Exercise and Physical Activity for PCOS

Regular exercise is a key component in managing PCOS, improving insulin sensitivity, and maintaining overall health. Here's how to incorporate exercise and physical activity effectively:

1. Benefits of Exercise for PCOS

Improves Insulin Sensitivity: Helps regulate blood sugar levels and reduce insulin resistance.

Supports Weight Management: Aids in maintaining a healthy weight, which can alleviate PCOS symptoms.

Reduces Androgen Levels: May help lower excess testosterone levels and improve hormonal balance.

Enhances Mood and Reduces Stress: Regular
physical activity can improve mood and reduce
anxiety and depression.

2.Types of Exercise

Aerobic Exercise: Increases cardiovascular health
and burns calories. Aim for at least 150 minutes per
week of moderate-intensity activities like brisk
walking, cycling, or swimming.

Strength Training: Builds muscle mass and boosts
metabolism. Include exercises like weight lifting,
resistance bands, or bodyweight exercises (e.g.,
squats, lunges) 2-3 times a week.

Flexibility and Balance: Improves overall mobility
and reduces injury risk. Incorporate stretching,
yoga, or Pilates into your routine 2-3 times a week.

3. Designing an Exercise Routine

Set Realistic Goals: Start with achievable goals
and gradually increase intensity and duration.

Create a Schedule: Plan your workouts around
your daily routine to ensure consistency.

Mix It Up: Combine different types of exercise to
keep your routine varied and engaging.

4. Tips for Success

Find Activities You Enjoy: Choose exercises that you find fun and motivating to increase adherence.

Listen to Your Body: Adjust the intensity and type of exercise based on how you feel and any physical limitations.

Stay Consistent: Aim for at least 30 minutes of physical activity most days of the week.

5. Example Weekly Exercise Plan

Monday:
30 minutes of brisk walking or jogging
20 minutes of strength training (e.g., upper body workout)

Tuesday:
30 minutes of yoga or stretching

Wednesday:
30 minutes of cycling or swimming
20 minutes of strength training (e.g., lower body workout)

Thursday:
30 minutes of brisk walking or light jogging
15 minutes of core exercises (e.g., planks, leg raises)

Friday:

30 minutes of dancing or a fitness class
15 minutes of stretching

Saturday:
45 minutes of outdoor activity (e.g., hiking, biking)

Sunday:
Rest day or gentle stretching

6. Staying Motivated

Track Progress: Keep a journal or use an app to monitor your workouts and improvements.

Set Achievable Milestones: Celebrate small victories and progress to stay motivated.

Exercise with a Partner: Find a workout buddy for support and accountability.

Incorporating regular exercise into your routine can significantly impact your PCOS management and overall well-being. Aim to find a balance that works for you and enjoy the benefits of physical activity.

Stress Management Techniques

Effective stress management is crucial for overall health and well-being, particularly for those managing PCOS, as stress can exacerbate symptoms. Here are various techniques to help manage and reduce stress:

1.Mindfulness and Meditation

Practice Mindfulness: Focus on the present moment without judgment. Techniques include mindful breathing, body scan, and mindful walking.

Try Meditation: Spend a few minutes each day meditating to calm the mind and reduce stress. Apps like Headspace or Calm can be helpful.

2.Physical Activity

Regular Exercise: Engage in activities like walking, yoga, or swimming to reduce stress hormones and improve mood.

Gentle Movement: Incorporate relaxation-focused exercises such as Tai Chi or gentle stretching.

3.Healthy Lifestyle Choices

Balanced Diet: Eat a nutritious diet rich in whole foods, which can positively impact stress levels and overall health.

Adequate Sleep: Aim for 7-9 hours of quality sleep per night to help regulate stress and support overall well-being.

Hydration: Drink plenty of water to stay hydrated and support bodily functions.

4.Relaxation Techniques

Deep Breathing: Practice deep, slow breathing to activate the body's relaxation response. Try the 4-7-8 breathing technique (inhale for 4 seconds, hold for 7 seconds, exhale for 8 seconds).

Progressive Muscle Relaxation: Tense and then slowly relax each muscle group to alleviate physical tension.

5.Time Management

Prioritize Tasks: Create a to-do list and prioritize tasks to manage your workload effectively.

Break Tasks into Smaller Steps: Break larger tasks into manageable steps to reduce overwhelm.

6.Social Support

Connect with Others: Spend time with friends and family to build a support network.

Seek Professional Help: Consider therapy or counseling if stress becomes overwhelming or persistent.

7.Hobbies and Interests

Engage in Enjoyable Activities: Dedicate time to hobbies or activities that you find enjoyable and relaxing.

Creative Outlets: Try activities such as painting, writing, or playing music to express yourself and reduce stress.

8.Mind-Body Techniques

Yoga: Practice yoga to combine physical movement, breath control, and relaxation for stress reduction.

Tai Chi: This gentle martial art focuses on slow, deliberate movements and deep breathing.

9.Setting Boundaries

Learn to Say No: Set boundaries and avoid overcommitting to reduce stress.

Balance Work and Personal Life: Make time for relaxation and self-care alongside work and other responsibilities.

10.Positive Thinking

Practice Gratitude: Keep a gratitude journal and regularly reflect on positive aspects of your life.

Challenge Negative Thoughts: Reframe negative thinking patterns to focus on positive outcomes and solutions.

Incorporating these stress management techniques into your daily routine can help reduce stress and improve overall well-being. It's important to find what works best for you and to integrate these practices consistently into your life.

Sleep and Its Impact on PCOS

Sleep plays a crucial role in managing PCOS and overall health. Poor sleep can exacerbate PCOS symptoms, while good sleep hygiene can support better hormonal balance and metabolic health.

Impact of Poor Sleep on PCOS

1.Hormonal Imbalance:

Insulin Resistance: Inadequate sleep can worsen insulin resistance, leading to higher blood sugar levels and increased risk of type 2 diabetes.

Elevated Androgens: Poor sleep may lead to higher levels of androgens (male hormones), which can worsen symptoms like acne and excessive hair growth.

2.Weight Gain:

Increased Appetite: Lack of sleep can affect hunger hormones (ghrelin and leptin), leading to increased appetite and weight gain.

Altered Metabolism: Disrupted sleep can impact the body's ability to metabolize carbohydrates and fats effectively.

3.Mood and Stress:

Increased Stress: Poor sleep can elevate stress levels, which can further exacerbate PCOS symptoms and lead to mood swings, anxiety, and depression.

Reduced Cognitive Function: Sleep deprivation can impair cognitive function and emotional regulation, affecting overall well-being.

4.Immune System Function:

Weakened Immunity: Chronic poor sleep can weaken the immune system, making the body more susceptible to infections and inflammation.

Benefits of Good Sleep for PCOS

1.Improved Insulin Sensitivity:

Better Glucose Control: Adequate sleep helps regulate blood sugar levels and improves insulin sensitivity, reducing the risk of developing type 2 diabetes.

2.Balanced Hormones:

Lower Androgen Levels: Quality sleep helps balance hormone levels, potentially reducing symptoms such as acne and hirsutism.

Stable Mood: Good sleep supports emotional well-being and helps manage stress more effectively.

3.Weight Management:

Controlled Appetite: Proper sleep helps regulate hunger hormones, supporting healthier eating habits and weight management.

4.Enhanced Overall Health:

Improved Immune Function: Sufficient sleep strengthens the immune system, helping to manage inflammation and support overall health.

Tips for Improving Sleep Quality

1. Maintain a Regular Sleep Schedule:

Consistent Bedtime: Go to bed and wake up at the same time every day, even on weekends.

2.Create a Relaxing Bedtime Routine:

Wind Down: Engage in calming activities before bed, such as reading, gentle stretching, or taking a warm bath.

3.Optimize Sleep Environment:

Comfortable Setting: Ensure your bedroom is cool, dark, and quiet. Invest in a comfortable mattress and pillows.

4.Limit Screen Time:

Reduce Blue Light Exposure: Avoid screens (phones, computers, TVs) at least an hour before bedtime to prevent disruptions to your sleep cycle.

5.Watch Your Diet:

Avoid Caffeine and Heavy Meals: Limit caffeine and large meals close to bedtime, as they can interfere with sleep.

6.Get Regular Exercise:

Active Lifestyle: Engage in regular physical activity, but avoid vigorous exercise close to bedtime.

7.Manage Stress:

Relaxation Techniques: Practice stress-reducing
activities such as meditation, deep breathing, or
yoga.

Incorporating these sleep strategies into your
routine can help manage PCOS symptoms and
improve your overall quality of life. Prioritizing good
sleep hygiene is essential for achieving better
hormonal balance and overall health.

CONCLUSION

Effectively managing PCOS requires a comprehensive approach that includes balanced nutrition, regular exercise, stress management, and good sleep hygiene. By understanding the role of diet in controlling symptoms, incorporating physical activity, and addressing stress and sleep, you can significantly improve your quality of life and overall health.

Key Takeaways:

Balanced Diet: Focus on low-glycemic, anti-inflammatory foods to help manage insulin resistance and hormonal imbalances associated with PCOS.

Regular Exercise: Incorporate a mix of aerobic, strength, and flexibility exercises to support metabolic health, improve insulin sensitivity, and enhance overall well-being.

Stress Management: Utilize techniques such as mindfulness, relaxation exercises, and social support to reduce stress and its impact on PCOS symptoms.

Quality Sleep: Prioritize good sleep hygiene to regulate hormones, manage weight, and support overall health.

By integrating these strategies into your daily routine, you can take control of PCOS and work towards a healthier, more balanced life. Remember that consistency and a personalized approach are key to finding what works best for you. If needed, consult with healthcare professionals to tailor strategies to your specific needs and circumstances.

Final Thoughts and Encouragement

Embarking on a journey to manage PCOS can be both empowering and challenging. Remember that you are not alone in this, and each step you take towards better health is a victory.

Embrace Your Journey:

Personalize Your Approach: Understand that managing PCOS is a personal journey. What works for one person may not work for another, so be patient and find what suits you best.

Celebrate Small Wins: Acknowledge and celebrate every positive change, no matter how small.

Progress is progress, and every step forward is significant.

Stay Informed and Empowered:

Educate Yourself: Continue learning about PCOS and its management. Knowledge empowers you to make informed choices and advocate for your health.

Seek Support: Connect with healthcare professionals, support groups, or online communities. Sharing experiences and seeking guidance can provide valuable support and encouragement.

Maintain a Positive Outlook:

Focus on Your Strengths: Emphasize your achievements and strengths rather than solely focusing on challenges. A positive mindset can greatly influence your well-being and motivation.

Practice Self-Care: Prioritize self-care and make time for activities that bring you joy and relaxation. Your well-being is a priority.

Commit to Your Health:

Consistency is Key: Adopting and maintaining healthy habits takes time and persistence. Stay committed to your health goals, and remember that every effort counts.

Adapt and Adjust: Be flexible and open to adjusting your approach as needed. Life circumstances and needs can change, and adapting your strategies can help you stay on track.

Managing PCOS is a journey of self-discovery and growth. By making informed choices and caring for yourself holistically, you can navigate this journey with resilience and optimism. Embrace each day with hope and confidence, knowing that you have the power to make positive changes for your health and well-being.

www.ingramcontent.com/pod-product-compliance
Lightning Source LLC
Chambersburg PA
CBHW070846250726
48662CB00003B/1394